Sanricu
A Collection of Unknown
Common Diseases in the
21st Century
A Disease May Be Rare But
Hope Should Not Be

Eleanor Christianson

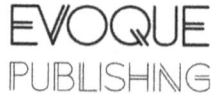

SANRICU

By ELEANOR CHRISTIANSON

Cover Design: Evoque Publishing

Interior Design: Evoque Publishing

Publisher: Evoque Publishing

Editor: Christine Joy A. Soliano

---

1. Health
2. Wellness
3. Treatment
4. History
5. Science
6. Education & Reference

Printed in London, United Kingdom

TABLE OF CONTENTS

Introduction

Life has always been described as harsh by the majority of people. In fact, contentment remains a prime need for all. The rich will always have predicaments, while the poor struggles with going through bare essentials. For people in their autumn years, pondering occurs more time and again.

"Is there more to life than what I am experiencing now?"

"Will I spend the remaining days of my existence working for survival?"

"Have all the excellence of my youth faded with time?"

What makes it worse is the emergence of various unknown, yet common, ailments in this century. These give ways to more questions in the minds of many people, irrespective of gender, culture, and religion. For these reasons, this book was created.

Although much knowledge is imparted in this book, it may not necessarily answer all your inner queries, especially concerning specific cures. Hence, it simply aims to provide you with a wider insight on the presence of these diseases and how it may affect the existence of the concerned individuals and their family.

The intention in writing this book is to share with you the present thrust of what goes in the life of an individual in general. As a non-fiction book, it seeks to share you some predicaments and how people may handle them. Once again, allow me to reiterate that this book may not be able to offer precise and instant solutions.

Instead, this book aims to add to your knowledge, to assist you to manage your unique situation. In addition, it seeks to strengthen your resolve and assist you to perceive the other life facets that you may have not given the correct importance.

For those afflicted by any of the maladies cited in this book, you will be able to see yourself and your life through the lens of a powerful microscope. You may get painful realizations in the process or feel relieved in knowing you are not alone in your individual quest.

As stated, life never promises the best for anyone. In its place, it poses a challenge that goes with your divine gift of choice. This freedom to choose makes you special and unique. The manner you go through life defines you and what matters most in your life. This book, therefore, serves as an evaluation of your today, so you can make the necessary modifications. Obviously, such adjustments are geared towards attaining a better tomorrow.

Ultimately, you could move on to that inevitable date when you embrace peace with no reluctance or regret. You can then let go of your remaining moments, knowing that you have done all that was needed.

Chapter 1: 21st Century Trends

It is expected that, through the passing of time, the world population will consistently mushroom. Unavoidably, the reserves of the planet will be depleted and alterations will occur. The epic on population no longer concerns development, but now focuses on communal decline, slow-moving growth, senior folks exceeding the number of the young people, and preference for residing in metropolitan areas.

For growth, it is where every trend occurs, as well as how they impact one another. The spitting image of several countries having high growth in population—almost all in Africa—exists as several countries have falling numbers of people in transitioning countries.

These extremes within population tendencies create powerful imperatives in such countries, as well as amongst countries that favor development projections with respect to social security nets, work conditions, fitness and care essentials, and a multitude of similar issues.

Demographic drifts between these extremes stay apparent within areas of the globe today. Increasing statistics of mid and equally low-income nations are suffering slow growth in population, whereas others have attained a productiveness plateau on still-high rates of growth.

Moreover, the growth paths representing every demographic condition are different from one another. In addition, it does not fit much on the normal development trail conceived in the previous century. Let us consider some areas heavily affected by the increase in population in our world.

Infrastructure

Countries face tough options to create financing for different infrastructure types. Should educational institutions come foremost of all?

What about the water system and similar agricultural necessities to feed the population? And they could not ignore the value of highways, bridges and transportation facilities for trade.

Then there is communication, energy and so much more. There would always be a completion of the urgent prerequisites for equally private and public infrastructures. In addition, the growth percentage and age of the people help determine the primacies of these needs.

Poverty

Fertility options are extremely related towards economic issues. For instance, people having higher income are likely to possess fewer kids than those with lesser income.

Is this due to having extra income that reduces the longing to put up with children? Or, because possessing fewer children increases income through allowing additional time towards earning it? Could it take place because people with lower income in some nations cannot manage or don't have easy access towards family preparing methods?

Public funds

While the developing nations of the world are projected towards seeing rapid upsurges in their older population, they are usually in the right direction to encounter considerable financial growth. This includes the attendant developments in the way of life standards that the majority will not possess.

This indulgence of being rich prior to becoming older seems not the way for the modern world. The next wave of countries would need to get ready today for elevated costs connected with belonging to an old society, notably the great costs of health care and pension funds.

Certain countries already possess the profile of the demography of industrialized countries, but lack the financial stability. In addition, they also do not have the prosperity of advanced countries. These countries are Argentina, Uruguay, Latin America, Barbados, Chile, as well as Trinidad and Tobago. After 14 years, it is predicted that only undeveloped countries in the world would be those within Gulf States, Sub-Saharan Africa, Nepal, Bangladesh, and Pakistan.

For growing markets, a population getting old will start to take part in savings, which is frantically needed to for investments towards sustaining economic development. The nations that comprise another aging ripple lag behind the industrialized lands, in relation to the present and the future, estimated stages of capital creation.

Climate change

At the minimum, three trends in demography are pertinent to climate changes. These are:

1. Age arrangement transitions, besides attendant vicissitudes in eating patterns, that are a valid development for industrial countries and many crowded emerging nations, which by 2050 will possess age arrangements resembling that of the industrialized world;
2. Movement in population and upsurges in eating related to urban living; and,
3. In-place growth in population, a factor in emissions of greenhouse gas.

New studies suggest that population growing in equally developing and developed nations tend to play an extremely important part in worldwide emissions of greenhouse gas. What the guideline implications aimed might be perhaps a little less well-defined.

Migration

The center of the development and demography projects are on the migration from deprived countries towards richer countries and, on a smaller extent, towards other underprivileged countries. Statistics during 2005 showed that more or less 60 million individuals moved residence from a lesser developed country to a far developed one.

This is roughly equal to those who migrated from a less advanced country towards another lesser developed one. The yearly immigration percentage in America reached its topmost in the 19th century at 11.6 percent of population dropping to 0.4 percent. This number rose again towards four percent at the end of the century with the real immigrant's count in America estimated at about a million each year, the maximum ever.

Indeed, the changes brought about in this century are massive and cover almost all aspects of life. The factors discussed above, in relation to demographic changes, also give rise to social, educational, technological, mental and even physical alterations in humanity.

In the process, these changes brought about more alterations, including diseases that have become common, yet unknown to many. In the next chapters, we shall take a keener look at these illnesses and discuss probable coping means, if not cure, to each of them.

Chapter 2: Gulf War Syndrome

This exists as a sickness told by battle troupers within the 1991 Persian Gulf War typified by symptoms that involve birth imperfections and immune system disorders. It is not clear whether these indications were connected with the Gulf War job, or the happening of diseases in the war troupers is advanced than similar populations. Symptoms credited to this condition have been extensive, including insulin resistance, lingering fatigue, damage on muscle direction, headaches, nausea and balance deficiency, memory problems, joint and muscle pain, stomach ache, skin complications, and shortness of breathing.

While the root of this syndrome stays unknown, several theories were anthrax inoculations given towards the soldiers, the usage of worn-out uranium as weapons, and contact to biochemical weapons demolished in numerous bombings. There remains also some conjecture that it might be produced by an unidentified bacteria.

A noticeable condition affecting war experts is a bunch of pathologically-unexplained long-lasting symptoms that the Veterans Affairs (VA) calls as a continuing multi-symptom illness or diseases not diagnosed. In general, though, it is simply called as the Gulf War Syndrome (GWS) because warning signs vary far and wide.

In fact, Gulf War old-timers need not prove a link between their armed forces service with the illnesses to properly receive their disability benefit. The VA believes that certain enduring, unexplained signs exist for half a year or so as related towards Gulf War facility without pertaining to the cause.

However, these probable illnesses must appear during duty in force in the Southwest Asia sphere of armed forces operations, or through 31 December 2016, besides being 10 percent disabling at the minimum. These diseases include:

1. Chronic Fatigue Syndrome – a long-term condition of severe exhaustion not easily calmed by relaxation and is not directly caused by related conditions;
2. Fibromyalgia – a disorder characterized via widespread pain in the muscles. Other indicators may be insomnia, stiffness in the morning, headache, and memory difficulties; and,
3. Functional gastrointestinal disorders – a cluster of circumstances marked through chronic, if not recurrent, indications related towards any portion of the stomach. Take note that functional illnesses refer to an irregular operation of a body part, without a physical alteration within the soft tissues. Examples comprise irritable bowel syndrome (IBS), functional indigestion, and functional intestinal pain conditions.

Diseases with symptoms without a diagnosis, but impartial to, comprise:

- Abnormal loss in weight;
- Fatigue;
- Heart disease;
- Joint, muscle, and head pain;
- Menstrual complaints;
- Psychological and neurological problems;
- Skin disorders;
- Respiratory illnesses; and,
- Sleeping complaints.

The good news is that Gulf War old-timers may be qualified for many welfares provided by the VA, such as:

- Airborne risks registry;
- Health upkeep;
- Gulf War registry fitness examination;
- Open burn pit registry; and,
- Disability reimbursement for illnesses connected with rendering military work.

In fact, their survivors and dependents may also be entitled to benefits. Likewise noted, is the continuous research on illnesses of the Gulf War veterans. The VA and other scientists continue conducting research towards investigating how working in the Gulf War is interconnected to illnesses the veterans are experiencing. Research comprises:

1. Medicine to methodically review the proof for probable connections amid illnesses;
2. Multiple year health investigation of Gulf War veterans towards finding out the manner their fitness has modified through time;
3. Studies conducted by Injury Study Center and War Related Illness of the VA; and,
4. VA agreements with IOM or the Institute of Gulf War veterans and contact with environmental causes or pre-emptive medicine in service, as well as the finest treatments meant for these diseases.

So far, the known causes are:

- Sarin – a lethal nerve instrument same with what was used in the attacks of Tokyo passageway;
- Mustard fume – a sweltering agent that burns the lungs and flesh;
- Fallout of organic agents – issued during and after the joined bombardments of Iraqi biochemical warfare weapons facilities;
- Botulinum and anthrax toxoid inoculations – together with some other new vaccines forcibly directed to American troops as if they were guinea pigs;
- Exposure to a minimum of 21 possible reproductive toxic agents – possibly damaging them and their children in the future;
- Pyridostigmine bromide – an anti-nerve preventive medicine forcibly ordered on American soldiers. Its usage in concurrence with DEET pesticide may probably have been horrible;
- Fifteen germ war agents – like incognitus and mycoplasma fermentans, which poisons cells of humans and injures them; and,
- Depleted Uranium (DU) – this remained generally hidden from the knowledge of the public. This material is found in the British and American weapons and also in the armor used within the Gulf war. Hence, the civilians and troops were equally exposed towards weapons created from dangerous depleted uranium.

Take note that DU is the deadliest source of the GWS. It contains deadly nuclear surplus and is proficient in causing nearly all indications of the GWS.

Aside from the assistance provided by the VA, there also exists natural curative modalities for GWS, such as:

1. Homeopathy

Historically, this has established far effectiveness on many occasions than other medical systems within the handling and inhibition of illnesses, without the danger of damaging side results. In the 1849 American cholera epidemic, allopathic medication saw an average death percentage of 54 percent, whereas, homeopathic infirmaries had a recorded death ratio of just 3 percent.

Roughly, the same statistics hold factual for cholera in the 21st century. New epidemiological research shows homeopathic medicines as matching or exceeding standard inoculations in stopping the disease. At hand is information wherein populations nursed through homeopathic remedies following a contact had a perfect success rate, meaning no one treated had been sick. Depending on the symptom, examples of homeopathic remedies are:

a. Nausea and travel sickness

Olives help but it is not as good as **ginger**. It is traditionally consumed to cure nausea, although it also works quite better against air sickness.

To prepare ginger tea, just slice a little quantity of garden-fresh ginger, then steep it in newly boiled water for half a minute or so. Ginger is very strong, so sample it at steady intervals of half a minute. You can also consume half a teaspoon of newly grated ginger as a faster alternative, although this way may not be so elegant.

Additionally, you may use **black horehound** and **peppermint** as disclosed in a study conducted by the Maryland University Medical Center. These aromatic plants can be consumed as fluid extracts or desiccated extracts in tea, powder or capsules, tinctures,. To create a tea with dried peppermint, put a teaspoon of peppermint into a strainer. Then, place it in a mug of boiled water, without adding sweeteners. If you really need a bit of sweetness, you may drop a little liquid stevia in it.

Another outstanding technique to combat nausea is the **Emotional Freedom Technique (EFT)**. It steadies your delicate energy structure and relaxes your kinetic sensors. As a result, this calms your indications of nausea or motion sickness, as well as allowing you towards finally enjoying the blisses of traveling.

b. Eczema

A truly simple and cheap way towards relieving the token eczema itch is putting a **brine compress** above the prickly area. You will want to make use of a high-level quality organic salt—like the sea rock salt or the Himalayan salt. Simply create a mixture with hot water, immerse the compress, and then apply the pack over the involved area.

You might also want ensure your complexion is hydrated at the optimum. The use of skin ointments is not really recommended as the solution here. Instead, hydrate your complexion from within by eating high excellent, animal-based **omega-3 fatty acids** within your food regimen, such as krill oil.

It is also helpful to take a little **gamma linoleic acid**, naturally found in primrose oil. Take note that plant-based omega-3, such as hemp and flax seed, will not deliver the scientific benefit you need to lessen skin swelling and inflammation, although they are good omega-3 resources.

Additionally, allergies in food play a huge role within eczema. The highly common transgressing agent exists as gluten or wheat. Hence, avoiding it is an astute first initiative. Staying away from grains would also decrease the sugar content in your body, which would normalize your levels of insulin and bring down any skin inflammatory condition. Other usual allergens involve eggs and milk.

Finally, vitamin D from **sunlight** can become your bosom friend whenever managing eczema, psoriasis, and other conditions of the skin. Ideally, you would want to obtain vitamin D from a suitable sunshine contact because ultraviolet ray radiation upon your complexion will not absorb vitamin D and help reinstate optimal function of the skin.

High quantities of ultraviolet ray exposure straight on the affected portion of the skin would greatly enhance the excellence of the skin, but be careful of getting too much ultraviolet ray exposure or it will cause sunburn. If you cannot get ample amounts of sunlight during winter, a lofty quality and safe treating bed will suffice. A harmless **tanning bed** provides the enhanced forms of UVB and UVA wavelengths, deprived of the dangerous exposure to EMF.

c. Headache

If you are prone to having headaches, it would be best to assess your way of life to know the cause. There are many kinds of headaches, with each having its individual set of causes. In the wide-ranging headaches not due to poor posture or tension, avoiding gluten, grains, sugar, additives, and fluids altogether, except for **water**, seems particularly useful.

Also, one more common kind is a migraine. Those experiencing recurring migraines would likewise do fine heeding this recommendation. Stay on this plan for some time because dietary alterations take an interval to be effective. In line with this, studies disclosed its roots from too much consumption of artificial or raw sugar and aspartame.

d. Sore throat and upper lung infections

There is a pile of proof disclosing **vitamin D** having a fundamental role in your immunity. Supporting optimal levels of this vitamin is your primary defense to counter infections of any kind, including those in the upper respiratory system. The deficiency of this vitamin during winter, wherein the body manufactures as a response to sunshine, has been associated with the cyclical increase in flu and colds. Studies have also suggested a link between vitamin D deficiency and a bigger risk of infections in the respiratory system.

Another truly inexpensive and simple treatment that is surprisingly applicable hostile to upper respiratory diseases is the **hydrogen peroxide (H_2O_2)**. Numerous patients experienced remarkable outcomes in curing flu and colds within 14 hours after being administered a couple of drops of 3 percent H_2O_2 into every ear.

This bottled solution is available at all drug stores for a few dollars. When you try this, you would normally hear a bit of bubbling and perhaps be aware of a small stinging feeling. You have to wait till these sensations subside, which usually would take around less than 10 minutes, and then draw off the excess solution from each ear onto a paper hankie.

To manage a sore throat, use **uncooked honey**. Take note that the most of the honey sold in America is extremely refined or processed, which, similar to most refined foodstuffs, can encourage diseases and can even damage your fitness, instead of helping.

Remember that **lemon** promotes the well-being of humans by rapidly alkalizing the body, while honey kills any microorganism. Therefore, this remains a faultless choice for a fast cough medicine.

Here is an easy recipe utilizing all organic ingredients for a cough. Simply take a **lemon,** place it in a pan with water, and simmer it for three minutes towards softening it and killing any microbes it may have on its skin, then let it cool. Next, put **two cups of fresh honey** inside another pan atop a stove using the smallest amount of fire. Slice the lemon, mix it with the heated honey, and warm it for an hour. Drain the mixture, get rid of any seed, and allow it to cool. Put the brew in a bottle with cover and keep it in the fridge for use within the next two months. Make sure to throw any unused mixture after two months and replace it with a fresh brew.

As for the amount of intake, take half a teaspoon of the brew for a child weighing a maximum of 25 pounds, and double the dose for children weighing 50 pounds. For adults, the dosage is one tablespoon. Take this every six hours.

2. Transfer issues and immunity

Health is directly affected by the immunity of the specific individual. The start of nearly all communicable and wasting disease remains preceded, if not accompanied, via the inadequate resistant response. With increasing concerns about the risks of immunizations and antibiotic-resistant organisms, a newfangled weapon to counter disease stands sorely required.

Transfer issues are, based on almost half a century of study, highly helpful with the absence of side results. **Glutathione,** a chief antioxidant, is a salient line of protection against oxidative stress, diseases, radiation, toxins, pollutants, and viruses. Without it, the liver becomes overwhelmed by the buildup of contaminants, resulting in organ collapse and demise.

The glutathione level in the cells stands as a predictor of the length of time people live. Its mystery lies in sulfur chemical it holds. Sulfur exists as a tacky, smelly particle that acts similar to a fly paper. Thus, all bad stuff in the human body stick onto it, counting toxins and free radicals, such as mercury, besides other thick metals.

Normally it is manufactured and recycled within the physique, except at the time a load of toxic substances become so great. Nonetheless, you could do numerous things towards increasing this normal, yet critical, tiny part in the body. Starting today, you can boost your glutathione within your body by:

a. Consuming food rich in sulfur

The major foods are onions, garlic, and cruciferous veggies such as watercress, cabbage, kale, broccoli, collards, cauliflower, and much more.

b. Trying whey protein

This exists as a great resource of amino acid and cysteine building blocks for glutathione fusion. The whey protein, however, must be made from natural proteins. Hence, choose untreated and unprocessed milk that has no antibiotics, hormones, and pesticides.

c. Exercising

This boosts glutathione intensities and, in turn, improves your immunity and detoxification while enhancing the antioxidant fortifications of the body. Start developing a 30-minute daily exercise, such as jogging, walking or playing various athletic games. Strength drills of 20 minutes, undertaken thrice weekly, stays also beneficial.

d. Taking supplements that support glutathione production

Besides consuming fish oil and a multivitamin, support your glutathione intensities with fresh fruits and vegetables, high-quality whey protein, raw milk and eggs, red and organ meats, sea foods, and organic turmeric, while reducing stress.

3. Detoxification

Ignite the internal curing force of the body by eliminating toxins. However, the quickest way towards restoring wellness is stopping toxins in the body. Then, this should be followed by giving the physique the nutrition it needs towards repairing and rebuilding itself. You can do this through:

a. Replacing one meal every day using a cleansing smoothie

When it concerns detoxifying the body naturally, substituting a meal with a smoothie is a good move. For instance, the first or last meal of the day can be a fruit or vegetable smoothie. This is just a slight diet modification that will not cause your body any damage.

In fact, it is an excellent means of freeing yourself of substances that the body does not really need. And rather than drinking a store-sold concoction or enhanced drink, just have homemade smoothies of natural fruits and vegetables that cleanses the body properly. This helps with losing weight and keeps digestion functioning in the manner it must.

b. Relying on organic foodstuffs whenever possible

While you do not really need to consume only natural foods, there are certain staples where these stay a must. Thus, stay away from foods that may contain preservatives and pesticides. The easiest rule to follow is eating organic only when you have to eat the skin or the exterior part of the vegetable or fruit. Thus, when it comes to strawberries, tomatoes, apples and pears, eat organic produce.

c. Getting a wholesome and strong massage

Take note that massage is not just a calming luxury, but also a noble way of cleansing the physique. It is all within the kind of massage that you select and the manner that you utilize this towards improving your fitness and life. Therefore, if you want to get rid of contaminants in your body, you unquestionably have to obtain an intense bodywork that concentrates greatly on the stress points in the physique. A conventional Swedish kneading is beneficial, but more forceful and intensive massage, such as a Thai, Ventusa, Hilot or Sports massage, can function better.

d. Drinking a lot of water

If there exists something that naturally and easily helps you towards detoxifying your physique, it is definitely clean water. Most often, we even think that we are drinking ample enough of water daily, but do you really monitor the quantity of water you drink each day?

The minimum is eight glasses of around 8 oz. of water to assist your body get rid of toxins easily. Proper intake of water can definitely contribute towards having a clearer complexion, respiration, digestion, and proper function of organs besides having a highly effective circulation.

e. Replacing coffee with tea

A bit of caffeine is okay, but be cautious about the quantity you drink throughout the day. After a mug of coffee, switch to green tea for the rest of the day. Green tea produces vital antioxidants that the body demands in a natural way. It submits a little caffeine support to your body that helps you get started the same way coffee does before lunch.

The Gulf War Syndrome is a sad aftermath of wars. It can be a devastating experience for the veteran and his family. Wars occur for many reasons that we would rather not take up in this book. What can be a sad realization is, upon engaging in wars, people stand more to lose than gain.

Coming home alive is great for our soldiers, but what people do not know is that the battle does not end for these brave veterans. Even amidst the company of their loved ones, they remain fighting an inner battle, coping with traumatic experiences, and living up to the expectations of society.

Basically, this book is a tribute to all our veterans and a simple reminder to all to support them in their recovery. Our soldiers stepped forward to protect us when needed. Then, it is proper that we return this service with sincere understanding, compassion and support.

Chapter 3: 20th Century Disease

The 20th Century Disease exists as described by way of a lingering condition typified by harmful effects from contact with low chemical levels in state-of-the-art human situations. Suspected materials include petroleum and scented products, smoke, synthetic fabrics, pesticides, paints, and plastics.

However, the strange thing is that blinded tests have disclosed that patients with MCS do not really react towards chemicals. Instead, they react within tests not blinded especially when they feel exposed towards a cause. The origin of this disease remains unknown and was the emphasis of the unusual 1995 movie entitled "Safe," which featured Julianne Moore.

Also referred to as a total aversion syndrome, it is a disorder attributed towards allergic reaction to the setting. Sometimes, it may be found to be so grave that the afflicted person is incapacitated to live in the world today. Although popular mass media often carry tales about it, it does not contain much scientific writing.

It remains diagnosed through clinical environmentalists, which uphold, together with other concepts, that vulnerable individuals go through a burden in attacks by non-natural materials within the situation. The afflicted people usually possess multiple ill-defined symptoms with no biological cause found.

Nonetheless, they forcefully resist seeing a psychiatrist as they ascribe their indications to hypersensitivity. In fact, a set of 18 people purportedly afflicted with this disease was subjected to a school psychiatric session. Almost all of them owned a lengthy history of consultations with physicians, although their warning signs were typical of some well-known psychological disorders.

The histories, as well as management of three cases in the set, were eventually presented. It revealed that, although these three patients might have been found atypical as they had far severe psychiatric symptoms, the involvement shows that a psychological diagnosis must be taken up.

History

MCS first stood as a separate disease in 1950 by Theron G. Randolph. After 15 years, Randolph created the Society for Clinical Ecology, an association to indorse his thoughts about signs described by patients. As a result, clinical ecology emerged by way of an unofficial medical field.

Nineteen years later, the organization changed its designation to American Academy of Environmental Medicine. After six years, the organization, with its continued existence, noted through fibromyalgia, chronic fatigue syndrome, and GWS. The US EPA, American Lung Association, and American Consumer Product Safety Commission then published a pamphlet on interior air contamination that discussed MCS and other topics.

Symptoms

Symptoms vary in harshness, from slight to incapacitating. They are normal but unclear and general for a condition. The highly common symptoms are fatigue, short-term problems in memory, difficulty in concentrating, and muscular pain. An incomplete list of similar symptoms reported by patients attributed to this disease include:

- Difficulty in inhaling and exhaling;
- Pain in the abdomen, throat, head, and chest;
- Skin inflammation;
- Neurological indicators, such as restless leg syndrome, weakness, nerve discomfort, pins-and-needles sensation, and trembling;
- Tendonitis;
- Seizures;
- Visual disorders, like the halo effect, blurring, and focusing inability;
- Anxiety;
- Panic or anger;

- Sleep problems;
- Suppression of the immune structure;
- Digestive complications;
- Nausea;
- Indigestion or heartburn;
- Vomiting;
- Diarrhea;
- Joint tenderness;
- Vertigo or dizziness;
- Abnormal sharp sense of smelling;
- Sensitivity towards natural herbal or pine fragrance;
- Dry mouth and eyes; and,
- Overactive urinary bladder.

Causes

There exists no definite consensus representing the reasons of the warning signs of this disease. In 2007, a dissertation by the National Institute of Environmental Health Sciences defined it as a lingering, recurring ailment caused by the inability of a person to endure an ecological chemical or a kind of external chemical.

Some hypotheses were proposed regarding extreme sensitiveness to small concentrations of specific chemicals. The difference between bodily and mental causes are often hard to examine, and it remains particularly thought-provoking for MCS because numerous substances utilized to check for sensitiveness have a concentrated odor.

Odor prompts make dual blind research difficult for patients with MCS since scents could provoke a mental response or remember expectations, besides prior views. People having a diagnosis of MCS show no changes in blood pressure, indicator severity, or heartbeat when in contact with fresh air or towards solvents of extremely small concentrations.

Relationship to GWS

Several epidemiological and clinical studies performed in America and in the United Kingdom have scrutinized the happening of this disease in army personnel assigned in the late 19th century at the Persian Gulf. Several health symptoms and complaints reported by Gulf War veterans attributed towards the GWS are the same to those stated for the 20th Century Disease.

Hence, a cross-sectional epidemiological investigation based on population involving US Gulf War veterans, non-veterans, and reservists not deployed though enlisted both outside and during the Gulf War era, decided that the occurrence of MCS-kind symptoms within the Gulf War troupers was rather higher compared to the non-veterans.

After altering for possible confounding issues, such as sex, age, and army training, at hand was a strong association amidst individuals having MCS-type indicators and psychological treatment, be it through medication or therapy, before sent to war and, thus, before whatever possible deployment-related chemical contact.

The chances of recounting MCS were almost four times bigger for veterans of the Gulf War than non-veterans. These veterans possess an elevated rate of conditions with multiple symptoms when compared with military staff deployed elsewhere. Although it stood unexplained, GWS is not counted distinct from similar medically mysterious syndromes seen in noncombatant populations.

Treatment

In numerous studies, around 50 percent of the afflicted people who look for medical handling for MCS symptoms meet the standards for anxiety and depressive disorders. And since many persons eliminate complete food groups in trying to lessen symptoms, a whole evaluation of the diet of the patient is needed towards avoiding nutritional deficits.

Avoidance of chemicals

Holding off chemicals has scientifically been proven as the most successful MCS treatment. Avoidance just means removing exposures towards chemicals that cause adverse reactions. This cuts down the chemical burden on the body, specifically in the hepatic cleansing pathways of the skin.

Chemical circumvention begins with the frequently hidden biochemical cocktail within personal maintenance products, such as:

- Aftershave;
- All scented products, like bath items, shampoo, soaps and conditioner;
- Antibacterial wipes and hand sanitizer;
- Beauty products;
- Cologne;
- Cosmetics;
- Creams and lotions with fragrance;
- Deodorant;
- Hair gel, spray, mousse, and color;
- Nail polish and polish remover;
- Perfume;
- Shaving lotion;
- Skincare products; and,
- Toothpaste.

In its place, it would be best to use the following:

a. Aftershave – use hydrogen peroxide or witch hazel.
b. Cream and lotion - use scent-free versions or natural coconut oil, jojoba, and olive.
c. Deodorant – use natural salt crystal, hydrogen peroxide, or baking soda. A homemade blend I use is a 500-mL mixture of 70 percent disinfectant alcohol and a tablespoon of powdered alum. Just shake the blend before using through manual application.
d. Hair styling or coloring – use fresh lemon juice or natural aloe Vera gel. Personally, I use fresh coconut milk or oil. Meanwhile, all natural color variations and henna will do for hair coloring. For bleaching, peroxide can do the trick.
e. Scent – use essential oils, provided they're tolerated and fragrance-free products. Otherwise, eliminate fragrances completely.
f. Shampoo and conditioner - unscented variants, essential oils, baking soda, citric acid and vinegar may be used.

As for the rest, safer and unscented versions from health stores may be used, although going natural is the best for nail polish, polish removers and cosmetics.

Chemical-free housing

The inside environment is generally more polluted compared to the outside environment because of the far-reaching fragrances, cleaners, petrochemicals, thinners, and unstable organic mixtures found within building furnishing and materials. Therefore, a chemical-free home is significant for symptom reduction, functional enhancements, and improved ability towards withstanding exposures from inevitable generative forces in the overall environment. Here is a list of domestic home products that people with MCS must avoid:

- Air fresheners;
- All perfumed products, including aromatic washing detergents, cloth softener, besides dryer cloth, be it scented or otherwise;
- All-purpose cleaners and air sprays;
- Antibacterial trash and vacuum bags;
- Commercial and industrial substances;
- Disinfectant aerosols;
- Concentrated or powdered products, including scouring powder;
- Fertilizers;
- Pesticides and herbicides;
- Scented tallow candles and incense;
- Solvents; and
- Window cleaners

Instead, try using peroxide or white vinegar as a cloth softener after using borax, scent-free laundry soap or baking soda in the laundry. To freshen the air, you may also use white vinegar or simply open the windows to adequately ventilate your home. Another option is exposing tea bags or having fresh herbs inside your home.

Likewise, you can clean your windows and almost anything in your home with white vinegar. Borax or baking soda is also safe to use as an alternative for scouring powder. Meanwhile, applying peroxide and white vinegar can make a good disinfectant. As much as possible, use unscented home products.

Finally, borax can also be used as a pesticide, and using diatomaceous earth can save you the cost of needing herbicide. Additionally, treat weeds with salt and vinegar and just pull them manually when cleaning your garden or backyard.

Nutrient treatment

Recently, most competent physicians suggest forms of antioxidant and nutrient therapy for MCS patients. This is because MCS patients often endure faulty nutrient absorption. Either they are weak to take in sufficient food nutrients from what they consume or they require higher nutrient levels for detoxification progression.

It had also been discovered that increasing certain nutrient levels often decreases symptom harshness. Hence, strengthening antioxidants impart a defensive effect. The good news is that there remain many protocols and products available lately. It is also believed that the ailment is primarily triggered through volatile carbon-based solvent contact, organophosphorus or carbamate pesticide experience, organochlorine insecticide exposure, and pyrethroid insect killer exposure.

As a result, these triggers appear to increase the nitric oxide levels in the human body. Nitric oxide consequently acts with peroxynitrite, its oxidizing product, to uphold a spiteful cycle system, which stands responsible for ensuing MCS. Therefore, treatment must focus upon down-regulating this biological chemistry cycle and decrease symptoms through the agents, as follows:

1. A low dose of magnesium and copper
2. A modest dose of zinc
3. Acetyl L-carnitine
4. Alpha-Lipoic acid
5. Betaine or trimethylglycine
6. Carotenoids, counting alpha-carotene, lutein, and lycopene
7. Coenzyme Q10
8. Folic acid
9. Flavonoid resources: bilberry, cranberry, ginkgo biloba, and silymarin extract
10. Green tea extract
11. Magnesium by way of malate
12. Mixed organic tocopherols

13. Prescribed nebulized breathed in reduced glutathione
14. Protected vitamin C
15. Riboflavin 5'-Phosphate (FMN)
16. Selenium-grown yeast
17. Stipulated nebulized breathed in hydroxocobalamin
18. Vitamin B6 by way of pyridoxal phosphate

These nutrients could be bought separately without prescription, except when clearly indicated in the list. For additional information, it is best to consult your physician.

Sauna and detoxification treatments

There are numerous detoxification approaches that are helpful. However, testing must be done by a competent provider towards ruling out or curing pesticide and heavy metal intoxication. ***Chelation treatment*** may be taken into account in instances of recorded burdensome metal harmfulness.

Moreover, ***fasting*** must only be done with health supervision because the deployment of substances stored within body lipid during this process may lead to the aggravation of warning signs. Among the safe and sound methods of general detoxification suggested by skilled physicians is the ***sauna***.

This is a warmed up, insulated chamber intended for detoxification and cleansing. Saunas destroy environmental elements that remain stored within fatty cells through warming up the physique. As a result, it mobilizes chemicals from stored fat that are, eliminated through sweat. Here is the basic direction for a sauna treatment:

1. Set the temperature to an average of 173ºF for a sauna using traditional rocks or an average of 115ºF for far infrared sauna;
2. Shower before entering the sauna and drink a glass of cold water;
3. When in the sauna, sit on a mat or towel on the stall. With familiarity, you would learn whatever temperature functions best on your behalf. When this happens, adjust the heat accordingly;
4. Throw liquid on the rocks of the space heater to intensify the heat, and add moisture towards the ventilation within an old-fashioned sauna;

5. Rinse sweat by taking a shower after 15 minutes or when you sense the necessity to bring your temperature down. You may return for an extra 15 minutes, if preferred;
6. After the final round, take a bath to regain your usual body temperature and eliminate sweat;
7. Make sure to drink water during and after the sauna; and,
8. Frequent users of a sauna may also be interested in tri-salts towards replacing lost minerals and salts through sweating. Personally, I put a drop of peppermint essential oil to around 12 oz. of water for pouring water on the heated rocks of a traditional sauna. It never fails to provide me a relaxing detoxification experience!

Chapter 4: Microcephaly

Microcephaly is among the top 10 illnesses that are considered as the oddest of the weirdest rare sicknesses found in the 21st century. It is a rare nervous system condition wherein the head of a baby is pointedly smaller compared to that of babies of similar sex and age.

Sometimes discovered during delivery, microcephaly has generally been the mark of a brain growing abnormally inside the uterus or failure to grow as should be after nativity. Thus, children having microcephaly frequently have growth issues, especially when its cause is genetic by nature.

Causes

Microcephaly is caused by various environmental and genetic factors such as:

1. Cerebral anoxia – this occurs when there is a decreased oxygen quantity going to the head of the fetus due to certain pregnancy complications or delivery problems that could harm the supply of oxygen;
2. Chromosomal irregularities – example is the down syndrome;
3. Craniosynostosis – this refers to the early attachment of sutures or joints between the bone plates. As a result, the development of the brain and the skull of an infant is impaired. Treating such condition usually denotes a surgical procedure for the baby to disengage the attached bones;
4. Contact of the uterus with alcohol, drugs or several toxic substances – this endangers the fetus with possible brain abnormalities;

5. Fetal infections – such infections comprise toxoplasmosis, cyto-megalovirus, German measles, besides chickenpox;
6. Severe undernourishment – this occurs once the pregnant woman fails to receive enough food; and,
7. Uncontrolled phenylketonuria (PKU) within the mother – It is a biological flaw that hinders the ability of the body to process phe-nylalanine, an amino acid.

Reports stated that almost one in every 670,000 children has or will eventually possess a head that ceased growing. Consequently, their heads are smaller compared to average children. Moreover, more than 20,000 American children are subjected to this condition each year.

Symptoms

The initial microcephaly sign is a head with a size expressly smaller as compared to other babies of similar sex and age. The size of the head is cal-culated as the gap around the circumference or topmost part of the head of the child. Using consistent growth tables, the dimension is then compared with measurements of other children in percentages. Some babies possess small skulls, whose sizes fall low by way of the number one percentile.

In contrast, children having microcephaly, possess head sizes that no-tably measures below the mean, possibly equally below the number one percentile representing the sex and age of the baby. A baby, with an extra severe condition, may have a rearward-sloping temple.

Complications

This is an enduring condition without a cure for the moment, but at hand are certain positive advances that assist the kids to live an ideal life possible with the illness they face. Some children suffering from micro-cephaly possess normal aptitude and growth, even when their craniums continuously remain tiny for their gender and age. Depending on the rea-son and the harshness of the disease, complications might include difficul-ties in balance and coordination, facial alterations, hyperactivity, seizures, short body builds and developmental postponements, like those concern-ing mobility, speech and the mind.

Diagnosis and tests

To know whether a child developed microcephaly, the doctor will likely take a meticulous examination of the child's prenatal and natal history, and family history, as well as conducting a physical examination. He will gauge the perimeter of the head of the child, relate it to a development chart, then measure again and calculate the development at succeeding visits.

The head dimensions of the parents will also be taken to ascertain whether little heads are innate within the household. In several cases, especially if the development of the child is late, your physician may demand tests, like an MRI or CT scan of the head, and plasma tests to help determine the core delay cause.

Drugs and treatments

Generally, there is no cure for this ailment. But timely intervention through supportive treatments, similar to occupational and speech therapies, might help improve the development of the child and perk up the quality of his life. Apart from surgery representing craniosynostosis, there is generally the absence of treatment that would enlarge the head of the child or lessen the microcephaly complications.

Treatment concentrates on means to supervise the condition of the child. Early intervention packages that cover occupational, physical and speech therapy might help strengthen the abilities of the child. Your physician might suggest medication for certain microcephaly complications, like hyperactivity or seizures.

Support and coping

Upon learning that your kid has this condition, your feelings might consist of anger, anxiety, worry, sadness and remorse. You might not discern what to anticipate in the days to come, and end up worrying about the future of the child. The top antidote to alleviate worry and fear is support and information. Hence, you need to prepare by:

1. Finding a group of reliable professionals

You will need to create important choices about the treatment and education of your child. Thus, create a group of teachers, doctors, therapists, besides other specialists, who could help you assess the sources within your neighborhood and make clear federal and state programs for children having disabilities.

Medical departments your kid might need include general and developmental pediatrics, neurology, infectious diseases, genetic, psychology and ophthalmology.

1. Seeking families coping with similar issues

Your area might have care groups for parents of kids with growth-related disabilities. You may also try to locate online care groups.

Prevention

Finally, learning that your kid has this condition can bring about questions concerning the future bearing of children. Work alongside your physician to know the reason for the disorder. If it is in the genes, consider talking to a counselor specializing in genetics about the dangers of this condition in upcoming pregnancies.

Chapter 5:
Kuru and Creutzfeldt-Jakob Disease

Found exclusively within New Guinea in an upland ethnic group known as the Kuru, this degenerative disease is directly triggered off by eating human flesh or cannibalism, wherein the existing kinfolks of a dead family member consume the organs and body. More than a thousand people were identified to have perished within 1950 and 1960.

Most of them have been comatose after losing their ability to stand or eat. It is also recognized by way of the "Laughing Death" representing its eerie ability towards having those plagued to burst into impulsive frenzied laughter. It was discovered that the head began deteriorating like a cheese, which means holes started to appear all around the brain.

This affected the limbs, besides coherence, before passing away. Government restriction on eating flesh, however, has significantly decreased the happening of this illness. Creutzfeldt-Jakob disease (CJD), on the other hand, is known to cause dementia, and worse death. Its symptoms can appear like those of similar dementia-like cerebral disorders, like Alzheimer's, yet it usually advances much rapidly. This rare disease captured the attention of the public in the late 19th century when several people within the UK developed a variant CJD after consuming meat from a diseased cow.

Although grave, CJD exists as a rare disease. Worldwide, the present is a projected one circumstance CJD identified per a million persons every year, and more frequently in senior adults. CJD or Creutzfeldt-Jakob disease, including its other forms, fit a wide group of animals and humans by way of transmissible spongiform encephalopathies (TSE).

The designation originates from the soft holes, noticeable under an optical microscope, that grows in brain tissues. Its cause and that of other

TSEs are strange forms of prion, a protein type. Normally these are not dangerous, but once their shape alters, they turn infectious, besides harm common biological procedures.

Transmission

The danger of CJD stays low as the ailment cannot be passed on through sneezing or coughing, sexual intercourse or touching. Instead, it fosters in three modes:

1. Contamination
Limited people have acquired CJD through exposure to diseased human flesh during a health procedure, like a skin or cornea transplant. Also, due to standard disinfection methods not destroying irregularly shaped prions, a couple of people developed CJD from a brain surgical procedure with unclean instruments;

2. Genetic
In America, about 10% of the people afflicted with this disease have a history of the ailment in the family or have positive results for genetic metamorphosis related to CJD. This kind is termed by way of familial CJD; and,

3. Sporadically
Most individuals with traditional CJD grow the illness for no obvious reason. Termed sporadic, this kind of CJD explains the greater part of instances.

CJD cases correlated to curative procedures remain mentioned by way of iatrogenic CJD. Variants are linked principally to the consumption of beef contaminated with mad cow disease (BSE).

Symptoms

CJD is characterized by a fast mental decline, typically within a couple of months. Initial symptoms classically include:

1. Anxiety;
2. Blurred eyesight or no vision at all;

3. Depression;
4. Impaired judgment;
5. Insomnia;
6. Loss of memory;
7. Personality vicissitudes;
8. Speech difficulty;
9. Sudden irregular movements; and
10. Trouble with swallowing.

As the sickness progresses, symptoms in the mind worsen. Most persons eventually fall into unconsciousness. In addition, pneumonia, heart, and respiratory failure, or similar infections are generally the reasons for death, which usually takes place within 12 months.

For individuals with a rare variant of CJD, psychiatric warning signs may become more obvious at the onset, with the destruction of the capability to deliberate, reason and recall , developing far along the disease. Additionally, this modified form affects persons at a lesser age bracket than the classic disease. It also appears to possess a considerably longer period of more than a year.

Risk issues

Most instances of CJD, as previously mentioned, occur on behalf of unknown causes, and the absence of risk issues can be recognized. A couple of factors, however, seem to associate through different CJD kinds, such as:

1. Age
Its sporadic kind tends towards developing later within life, frequently around the age of 60. The start of the familial kind occurs somewhat earlier, while variant CJD has concerned people at a younger stage, usually within their approach of the age of 30.
2. Genetics
Folks having familial kind have a mutation in their genes that leads to the ailment. This is then inherited with an autosomal overriding fashion that means you have to receive only a reproduction of the changed gene from any parent towards developing the ailment.
If you possess the metamorphosis, the probability of transferring it to

your kids is 50 percent. Genetic examination in folks with variant CJD and iatrogenic suggests that getting identical reproductions of definite prion gene variants may enlarge your danger of having CJD when you are exposed towards contaminated flesh.

3. Contact with contaminated flesh

People who have received growth hormones from humans derived from the pituitary glands, or had tissue grafts that contain the dura mater, or even the brain may be endangered of iatrogenic CJD. The hazard of going down with a variety of CJD arising from consuming contaminated meat of a cow is hard to ascertain. Generally, if nations are effectively implementing community health actions, the peril is almost nonexistent.

Drugs and treatments

No operative treatment is present for CJD and its variations. Numerous medications have been tried, including antibiotics, antiviral therapies, and steroids, but none have shown any benefit. As a result, doctors concentrated on lessening pain, as well as other warning signs, and in making diseased people as contented as probable.

Prevention

There exists no renowned way towards preventing the sporadic kind of this disease. If you possess a history in the family of diseases on the nerves, you might benefit from consulting a counselor specializing in genetics, who could help you go through the dangers linked with the situation.

Meanwhile, hospitals and other health institutions adhere to explicit guidelines to avoid the iatrogenic kind of CJD. These procedures include:

1. Destruction of instruments used in the surgery of the nerves or brain of a person known, if not suspected, of having CJD;
2. Exclusive utilization of faux growth hormones of humans, instead of the type derived from pituitary glands of people; and,
3. Single-use sets for lumbar insertions or spinal punctures.

To ensure the protection of the blood supply, individuals with a possibility of contact with the disease or its variant are not eligible towards donating blood. This takes in people who:

1. Devoted at least five years since 1980 in France;
2. From 1980 and onwards, took blood transfusions in the United Kingdom;
3. Have a genetic relative diagnosed as afflicted with CJD;
4. Received a growth hormone from another person;
5. Had been injected with bovine insulin since 1980 and onwards;
6. Spent a minimum of 90 days in the UK from 1980 until 1996; and,
7. Went through a brain implant.

Moreover, the peril of going down with a variety of CJD within America remains enormously low. Just three instances have been recorded in America with the American Centers for Disease Control and Prevention. And these cases have strong proofs suggesting that they were obtained abroad, specifically two from the UK and the other from Saudi Arabia.

In the UK, where the bulk of CJD variant cases occurred, have less than 200 instances reported. CJD cases peaked amidst 1999 to 2000, and has been diminishing since. Furthermore, most nations have undertaken steps towards preventing BSE-infected meat from coming into the supply of food, including:

1. Constraints on specific parts of a cow for food processing;
2. Restriction on feeds to animals;
3. Strict processes in dealing with ailing animals;
4. Surveillance and examination methods aimed at tracking cow health; and,
5. Tight controls on cattle importation from nations where BSE is usual.

Chapter 6: Pica

Pica, likewise known by way of Magpie, is an eating disorder where individuals eat almost anything, with no discrimination, covering a period of more than a month. A zinc or iron deficiency exists attributed towards this ailment, where a maximum of 32 percent of afflicted individuals yearn for the far unusual stuff, including soap, feces of animals, cloth, soil, talcum powder, balls of hair, ice, paint, and many others.

Sadly, there is no remedy, but completing nutrient deficits may assist with this problem. Pica is the consumption of nonfood stuff that are inappropriate for the development of a person. Such craving is also not a part of any specific social norm or culture.

And persistently consuming these items could result in medical problems, like poisoning, bowel problems, and infections. Pica frequently occurs with supplementary disorders similar to an intellectual infirmity or autism spectrum disorder. Others are:

1. Rumination syndrome

This is a disorder characterized by repeated and persistent regurgitating of food followed by eating. It is not because of a health condition or an eating complaint, like binge-eating, bulimia or anorexia. Food stands returned and accumulated in the mouth deprived of gagging or nausea.

Sometimes, vomited food exists chewed and swallowed again or spewed out. This disorder can result in malnutrition when the food stays spat out or when the individual eats extensively less towards preventing the action. The rumination illness episode may be highly common for infants or with people having a cerebral disability.

2. Avoidance or restrictive eating disorder

This is typified by neglecting to attain the minimum everyday nutrition needs because of:

    a.   Avoiding food items with specific sensory traits, like texture, color, taste or smell;

    b.   Concerning about the end results of partaking food, similar to the fear of food obstruction. Its reasons, however, do not include avoidance for fear of obesity; and,

    c.   Simply having no interest in eating.

The malady can cause the significant loss in weight, inability to increase weight in childhood, and nutritional deficits that result in health troubles. Avoidance or restrictive eating disorder remains undiagnosed when warning signs are a portion of a supplementary eating sickness, similar to anorexia, or a fragment of a health problem or mental ailment.

Due to its influential pull, a consumption disorder could be tough to deal with or surmount on your own. Eating conditions can almost overrule your existence. If you are experiencing this problem, or think you might have a consumption disorder, it is best to seek professional medical assistance.

On the other hand, if you suspect a beloved to be afflicted with this condition, then do your best to urge him to find treatment. Unfortunately, numerous people having an eating complaint may not consider needing treatment. So, even when your beloved is not ready towards acknowledging having the food issue, you could inject the idea by stating your concern and your desire towards listening.

Be wary of eating habits and views that might signal unwholesome behavior and pressure from peers that can trigger disorders in eating. Warning signs that can indicate a disorder in consumption include:

    1.   Adopting an excessively restrictive vegan diet;
    2.   Eating more for a snack or meal than what is normal;
    3.   Excessive concern about eating healthy foods;
    4.   Expressing guilt, disgust, depression or shame about consumption habits;
    5.   Extreme exercise routines observed;

6. Frequent viewing of self in a mirror to check flaws in appearance;
7. Inducing puking to the point of having knuckles with calluses;
8. Leaving the dining table during meal time for toilet use;
9. Making home meals exclusively for personal consumption and not eating whatever family members eat;
10. Persistent complaining or worrying about excess weight and endless talks about weight loss;
11. Problems on losing tooth enamel, which may signify repeated spewing;
12. Repeatedly consuming large quantities of high-fat or sweet foods;
13. Secretly eating food;
14. Skipping meal times, if not coming up with excuses to skip a meal;
15. Use of herbal products, laxatives, or food supplements for losing weight; and,
16. Withdrawing from usual social events.

If you are troubled with your kid for possibly having a consumption disorder, it would be best to contact your doctor towards discussing your apprehensions. If required, you could get a recommendation from a trained mental specialist for management. Bear in mind that eating illnesses can cause a vast range of difficulties, some of which are even life-threatening. The severer or longer lasting the disorder, the more likely you will experience stern complications, like:

1. Anxiety and depression;
2. Death;
3. Problems concerning development and growth;
4. Relationship and social problems;
5. School and work issues;
6. Significant health difficulties, such as bowel obstruction, infection, and dental injury;
7. Substance abuse or disorder in using substances; and,
8. Suicidal behavior or thoughts.

Conclusion

The featured diseases in this book are but a few of the numerous rare diseases that ranges from the cannibalism Kuru to countless allergies. Be aware, too, that there are common diseases that are now moving to rarity. Moreover, there are others that have been nurtured as a result of genetic changes and profane habits.

In fact, countless of these diseases exist not simply infrequent, but likewise fantastically strange and seem to be possible only in one's imagination. So, let me ask you? What is the supreme bizarre illness for you? If you wish to read more on this topic, please do let me know.

We can always come up with a sequel to this book. For now, how about pondering on these rare and incurable diseases? What do you think is its essence in life? For me, it affirms the steadfastness of change and reiterates the need for people to constantly modify to meet the results of these changes.

Most of all, I look at these events as a challenge for mankind to hold on to faith, that despite what may be lacking today, there is hope for the days to come. And this hope will materialize for as long as there are people who believe and work for it. I pray every individual will do his share in keeping humanity healthy, however small or trivial the effort is.

Finally, if you have enjoyed this book, then I'd like to ask for a favour, would you be kind enough to leave a review for this book on Amazon? It'd be greatly appreciated!

To receive free updates on further releases from Eleanor Christianson and other material related to Health and Diseases from Evoque Publishing, sign up at the following url: www.evoquepublishing.com/signup

 https://www.facebook.com/EvoquePublishing

 https://twitter.com/EvoquePub

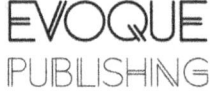